Natural Remedies for Headaches and Migraine
Top 50 Natural Headache Remedies Recipes for Beginners in Quick and Easy Steps

Rita Clark

Copyright © 2015 Rita Clark

All rights reserved.

ISBN-10: 1511485272
ISBN-13: 9781511485272

CONTENTS

Introduction	7
Part 1: Chamomile	9
Recipe 1: Basic and Effective Chamomile Tea	10
Recipe 2: Chamomile Herb Tea	11
Recipe 3: Lemon Balm Chamomile Tea	12
Recipe 4: Cinnamon Chamomile Tea Latte	13
Recipe 5: Chamomile Ginger Ice Tea	14
Recipe 6: Chamomile, Lavender Mint Ice Tea	15
Recipe 7: Chamomile Oil	16
Part 2: Ginger Tea	17
Recipe 8: Hot Ginger Tea	18
Recipe 9: Fresh and Spicy Ginger Tea	19
Recipe 10: Iced Ginger Tea	20
Recipe 11: Ginger Latte	21
Part 3: Banana	22
Recipe 12: Banana Whip	23
Recipe 13: Banana Dog Bites	24
Recipe 14: Creamy Banana Oatmeal	25
Recipe 15: Banana, Honey and Hazelnut Smoothie	26
Recipe 16: Banana Ginger Smoothie	27
Part 4: Potatoes	28
Recipe 17: Lemon Potatoes	29
Recipe 18: Honey and Dijon Potato Salad	30
Recipe 19: Potato Soup	31
Recipe 20: Mojo Potatoes	32
Recipe 21: Potato Pancakes	33
Part 5: Lavender	34
Recipe 22: Lavender Roasted Potatoes	34
Recipe 23: Hot Lavender Tea	35
Recipe 24: Pink Lemonade Lavender Sorbet	36
Recipe 25: Lavender infused Oil	37
Recipe 26: Lavender Honey Syrup	38
Part 6: Salads	39

Recipe 27: Romaine and Smoked Salmon Salad	40
Recipe 28: Apple and Carrot Salad with Ginger	41
Recipe 29: White Bean Asparagus Salad	42
Recipe 30: Grilled Salmon and Citrus Salad	43
Recipe 31: Avocado Watermelon Spinach Salad	44
Part 7: Juices and Smoothies	45
Recipe 32: The Green Juice	46
Recipe 33: Green Breakfast	47
Recipe 34: Veggie Blueberry	48
Recipe 35: Fresh Salsa	49
Recipe 36: Carrot and Aloe Juice	50
Recipe 37: Banana Milkshake	51
Recipe 38: Watermelon Migraine Buster Smoothie	52
Recipe 39: Grape and Green Smoothie	53
Recipe 40: Avocado Smoothie	54
Part 8: Cucumber	55
Recipe 41: Creamy Cucumber	56
Recipe 42: Cucumber and Avocado Sushi	57
Recipe 43: Cucumber Lemonade	58
Recipe 44: Cucumber Snack	59
Recipe 45: Cold Cucumber Soup	60
Part 9: Coffee	61
Recipe 46: Spicy Coffee	62
Recipe 47: Chocolate Cinnamon Coffee	63
Recipe 48: Banana Coffee Frappe	64
Recipe 49: Coffee Walnut Smoothie	65
Recipe 50: Ginger Coffee	66
Conclusion	67

Introduction

Headaches and migraines are defined as the pain in the head where you feel a tingling sensation of your head throbbing. You tend to feel disinterested in activities that you are doing as you are distracted by the constant hammering in your head. Sometimes, even your neck starts to pain, signaling the onslaught of a headache.

Headaches usually do not have any particular symptom. They can arise due to many reasons such as anxiety, fatigue, sleep deprivation, stress, or some viral infections. Even a minor tooth ache can sometimes lead to a headache.

Headaches can be classified as primary and secondary. In fact, there are more than 200 types of headaches; and a majority of them is harmless with only a few termed as life threatening.

At least 90% of the headaches are primary headaches with moderate to severe pains. Headaches are usually seen in the age bracket of 20 to 40 years with an average time span of six to eight hours depending upon the severity of the headache. However, it is not limited to any particular age group. Headaches can occur at any time, irrespective of the age of the person. At times you are also faced with 'never ending headaches' that cause you discomfort for days as well as lead you towards anxiety and fatigue.

Headaches can cause plenty of physical discomfort, starting from uneasiness to dullness. Due to this, a majority of the sufferers simply prefers to relax and stay away from work as much as possible or simply pop an over the counter available pill. Many drugs like Aspirin and other pain relievers are used, but these medications come with side effects. So if a person is chronic to headaches and migraines, popping a pill every now and then is certainly going to prove harmful in the long run. So what option a person has then? The answer to this would be natural harmless remedies. Even a person who suffers with headaches once in a while can look for natural remedies.

So what are you waiting for? Simply relax and start practicing these natural remedies to curb headaches and migraines.

Part 1: Chamomile

Chamomile is an herb that has been used as a medicine to curb many ailments since time immemorial. It is one of the safest herbs that is available naturally and can be used by humans. Chamomile is best used to curb headaches, especially stress related headaches and anxiety apart from many other ailments. Chamomile can be mixed with other herbs to generate the best results and to cure some specific ailments.

Recipe 1: Basic and Effective Chamomile Tea

Chamomile tea is highly recommended when you are suffering from headaches and migraine. Take a cup of this easy and highly recommended Chamomile tea to get relief from your headache.

Ingredients:

- Chamomile tea bag or loose-leaf chamomile tea
- 250ml of water
- Optional taste generators like honey, lemon or mint

Directions

Boil the water and add allow it to cool. Place the tea bag or loose-leaf tea into your mug and then add water to it. You need to make sure to allow the water to cool down for a few minutes. Chamomile tea tastes great when served with hot water and not boiling water. Allow the tea to steep for 5 to 10 minutes so as to bring out the flavor as well as the benefits. Afterwards, remove the tea bag and the Chamomile tea is ready to be served. You can then add the optional, if you desire. Honey tastes well and serves as a healthy and a delicious combination with Chamomile tea.

Recipe 2: Chamomile Herb Tea

Chamomile herb tea places a soothing and a calming effect around you and allows your headache to subside slowly and steadily.

Ingredients:

- One tablespoon fresh Chamomile flowers
- One cup of water
- Two thin slices of apples
- Honey

Directions

Rinse the Chamomile flowers thoroughly with cool water. Keep some water to boil. Take the apple slices, mash them and add it to the teapot. Also add the chamomile flowers and pour the boiling water into your teapot. Cover the pot and allow it to cool down from boiling to hot water. You can then add honey to enhance the taste.

This soothing hot cup of tea will calm your headache and migraine attack and will allow you to relax while having this delicious hot drink.

Recipe 3: Lemon Balm Chamomile Tea

Lemon balm as a combination with other herbs, especially with Chamomile flowers helps in reducing ailments like headaches. In this recipe, lemon balm is used along with Chamomile flowers and mixed to bring out the desired result to curb your headache and bring down the effect that migraine has on you. Lemon balm, as the name suggests, generates a mild lemon aroma that can be used for medicinal purposes.

Ingredients:

- 1 part dried chamomile flowers
- 1-2 parts dried lemon balm

Method:

Mix both the herbs well and store it in an airtight container for future use. Put two spoons of this mixture in an infuser and add it into hot or warm water as per your liking. This tea tastes best when taken hot.

Recipe 4: Cinnamon Chamomile Tea Latte

If you wish to have something different and unusual from the same tastes of chamomile tea, then this recipe is for you to taste. Not only does it taste great, but also helps in reducing the headache that is troubling you.

Ingredients:

- ¾ cup of water
- ¾ cup non-dairy milk, preferably cashew milk or almond milk
- 2 chamomile tea bags
- ¼ teaspoon ground cinnamon
- A pinch of salt and sugar for that perfect taste

Method:

Take a saucepan and fill it with a small quantity of water. Cover the pan and allow it to boil. Once the water is boiling, turn off the heat and add chamomile tea bags to it. Allow the tea to steep for at least 5-7 minutes (more, if you need the tea to be strong). After that, remove the tea bags and add the non-dairy milk, cinnamon, salt and sugar to it. Turn the heat on and allow the mixture to be hot but not boiling. Stir continuously while the mixture gets hot. Turn off the heat, pour the tea into your favorite cup and enjoy!

Recipe 5: Chamomile Ginger Ice Tea

A headache doesn't ask and occur. It simply happens without any prior notice and to beat that unwanted headache, sometimes it is good to prefer something cold than hot. Chamomile Ginger Ice tea is an alternative that is preferred when you are out for work under the hot sun and want to have something cool to ward off that irritating headache.

Ingredients:

- 2 cups of water
- 1 tablespoon grated and peeled ginger
- 1 tablespoon fresh lime juice
- 2 chamomile tea bags
- Ice
- 1-2 tablespoon honey

Method:

Boil the two cups of water in a saucepan. Once the water is boiled, remove the pan from the heat and add honey, ginger, chamomile tea bags and fresh lime juice to it. Allow it to steep for at least an hour. Once the mixture gets warm, pour it into a jar, discarding all the solids. Cover the jar and place it in the refrigerator, until it is extremely chilled. It is best to serve with some ice cubes.

Recipe 6: Chamomile, Lavender Mint Ice Tea

Lavender is extremely good for curing headaches. When used in a combination with chamomile, it gets all the more soothing and helpful in beating headaches and migraines.

Ingredients:

- Fresh mint leaves
- 1 tablespoon dried lavender for culinary use
- 1-2 chamomile tea bags

Method

Crush the mint leaves and add lavender and chamomile tea bags into a jar. Fill the jar with water and allow the mixture to refrigerate for at least 6 hours. You can then pour the mixture into a separate jar, removing all the solids from the mixture and enjoy this cool drink. The drink tastes all the better when served on the day after it is made.

Recipe 7: Chamomile Oil

Chamomile oil is useful for chronic recurring headache known as Migraine. The solution helps in reducing the pain and releases soothing fragrance that helps in fighting the migraine attack.

Ingredients:

- Dry chamomile flowers (1 cup)
- Sesame oil (5 drops)
- Vitamin E (1 teaspoon)
- Paper towel
- Glass jars with lid
- Cutting board
- Cheesecloth
- Sieve

Method:

Desiccate the chamomile flowers, clean them with water and place the flowers to dry out under the sun. Along with that, clean all the jars and make sure they are completely dry from within. Pour the sesame oil into the jar, leaving adequate space to add flowers into it. Add the flowers in the oil and make sure that the flowers are all soaked under the oil. Place the jar under the sunlight after placing the lid to it. You need to keep the jar under the sunlight for at least two weeks. After that, drain out the flowers using cheesecloth and add a few drops to vitamin E to the jar.

Chamomile oil is to be rubbed on the forehead and back for best results. It can also be inhaled.

Part 2: Ginger Tea

Ginger is known as an elixir for headaches and migraines. Ginger helps in reducing the pain and works as an anti-inflammatory agent. Once you get aware about the headache, it is time to have a cup of ginger tea before the pain escalates.

Recipe 8: Hot Ginger Tea

Nothing sounds better than a hot cup of ginger tea. Moreover, if you are suffering even from a mild headache, a hot cup of ginger tea will help you calm the pain and allow you to relax.

Ingredients:

- Pureed ginger (1 cup)
- Honey (1 cup)

Method:

Peel the necessary stash of fresh ginger completely and grate it finer into the form of a puree. Put this pureed ginger into a bowl and mix a cup of honey. Stir the mixture well. Place this mixture into a jar and store it in the fridge for cooling. To prepare a cup of hot ginger tea, take 2-3 tablespoon of the mixture and mix it with the boiling water. Your hot ginger tea is then ready to be tasted and served.

Recipe 9: Fresh and Spicy Ginger Tea

When the headache gives you ample amount of trouble, you need to beat it with a spicy ginger tea, which gives that extra amount of boost to fight the pain in your head.

Ingredients:

- 1 and half tablespoon peeled and chopped fresh ginger
- Half cup fresh lemon juice
- $1/4^{th}$ tablespoon cinnamon or one cinnamon stick
- Any sweetener, although Maple syrup is preferred
- A pinch of hot chili pepper

Method:

Take a cup of water along with ginger and blend it till the majority of the ginger is crushed. Pour this mixture into a pot of boiling water. Add cinnamon to the mixture. Reduce the heat to low once all the ingredients have been added to the mixture, including the sweetener. This will allow the mixture to steep slowly. You can then take this mixture and blend it for a much finer drink or can eat the initially small leftover pieces of ginger while taking a sip of the tea.

Recipe 10: Iced Ginger Tea

If you are looking out for some refreshing change from the hot ginger tea that you are having when caught with a headache, try the Iced Ginger Tea.

Ingredients:

- Half cup finely chopped ginger
- A few pods of cardamom
- A few cloves
- Black pepper
- Half teaspoon fennel seed

Method:

Boil the water in a pot and put each and every Ingredients into it. It is advisable to put at least 5 to 8 pieces of cardamom, cloves and black pepper. Keep the pot under the low flame for about thirty minutes and then turn off the heat. Keep the mixture in the pot overnight to allow steeping. Strain the mixture and pour it in a glass. Add almond milk or any milk as per your preferences along with sweetener and ice. Iced Ginger Tea is then ready to be served.

Recipe 11: Ginger Latte

The best way to enjoy a creamy, soothing, mildly sweet and perfectly gingerly is by having this Ginger Latte. It is a refreshing drink that can take the headache out of you.

Ingredients:

- 1 ½ cup water
- 1 cup chopped ginger
- 1 cup cane sugar
- 1 tablespoon ginger syrup
- 1 cup almond milk

Method:

To make the ginger syrup, place water, sugar and ginger into a pot to boil and keep on stirring till the sugar dissolves completely. Reduce the heat and continue cooking for another 30 to 40 minutes. Strain the mixture and place it in a bottle. Now to make the ginger latte, heat the almond milk and then add the ginger syrup to it. Sprinkle some cinnamon for a bit spicy taste.

Part 3: Banana

Bananas serve as a great source of food while curing headaches. Rich in magnesium and potassium, they help in relaxing your blood vessels and ease pain.

Recipe 12: Banana Whip

Banana whip is an energy drink as well as an excellent recipe to get rid of a hangover related to a headache. A glass of this drink definitely eases the pain and relieves you from headaches.

Ingredients:

- 2 medium sized bananas, peeled
- ¾ cup condensed milk
- 1 tablespoon vanilla extract
- 1 tablespoon chocolate chip
- A mixture of cinnamon and sugar

Method:

Cut the banana into small pieces and place them into a container. Add milk, vanilla and cinnamon sugar over the pieces. Blend the mixture till the banana pieces are finely pureed. Pour the mixture into small bowls as per your wish to intake and sprinkle with chocolate chips and cinnamon sugar for enhancing the taste.

Recipe 13: Banana Dog Bites

Banana Dog Bites is a refreshing recipe using banana that is high on energy as well as helps in relieving the pain caused due to headaches and migraines.

Ingredients:

- 2 peeled bananas
- ¼ cup peanut butter
- 2 tortillas

Method:

Apply peanut butter on one tortilla evenly. Place a banana on the edge of the tortilla. Roll it up nicely and slice it into equal halves. You can then heat the pieces for 30 to 40 seconds and have it hot.

Recipe 14: Creamy Banana Oatmeal

Oatmeal with banana serves as a perfect combination of healthy food along with capabilities to ease the headache that is nagging you. Oatmeal is a very delicious dish and can turn out to be even better with banana in the serving.

Ingredients:

- 1/3 cup of oats (depending upon the quantity you would like to eat)
- 1/3 cup of almond milk
- ½ mashed banana
- ½ tablespoon cinnamon
- ½ cup water
- Toppings – Nuts and others as per your liking

Method:

Pour the almond milk into a pan along with oats and place it on a medium heat. Put the mashed banana into the pan and keep stirring the mixture till the mixture turns out to be a bit creamier as banana melts. Sprinkle some cinnamon into the mixture as you stir. You need to ensure that the mixture doesn't turn out to be too sticky. While you stir the mixture, you can add toppings such as berries and nuts and cherish this amazing oatmeal dish.

Recipe 15: Banana, Honey and Hazelnut Smoothie

A banana smoothie is a go-to drink early in the morning, if you are suffering from severe headache. Just one glass is enough to restore order into your head by bringing normalcy and eliminating any traces of headache.

Ingredients:

- One peeled and sliced banana
- 250 ml of soya milk
- 1 tablespoon honey
- 1-2 tablespoon chopped hazelnuts
- Nutmeg

Method:

Put all the ingredients in a container and blend it until the mixture of banana, milk and grated nutmeg is smooth. Pour the blended mixture into a glass and top it with chopped hazelnuts. You can serve it with ice, if required.

Recipe 16: Banana Ginger Smoothie

Ginger, as we have seen, has great properties that can handle headaches and migraines. Combining it with a banana into a smoothie serves as an immediate relief from headaches and chronic migraines.

Ingredients:

- 1 cup milk
- 1 peeled banana
- ½ teaspoon peeled ginger, grated fine
- 1 tablespoon honey

Method:

Add all the ingredients and blend it until the mixture is smooth and a bit thick. Add honey if desired.

Part 4: Potatoes

Potatoes with their skin are best for relieving headaches. Potatoes are packed with potassium which helps in restoring balance in the head. Often the most neglected of the foods, potatoes have capabilities to eliminate headaches.

Recipe 17: Lemon Potatoes

Most of the times, potatoes are often regarded as one food instrumental in weight gain. But rarely do people understand that it is the oily and fried chips that are instrumental in weight gain and not potatoes in general. Lemon Potatoes is one such dish that helps in relieving headaches and also provides vital and much needed energy.

Ingredients:

- 3-4 even size potatoes
- 2 tablespoon olive oil
- ½ lemon
- Lemon juice
- Salt and black pepper

Method:

Cut each and every potato into 4-5 equal pieces, depending upon the size. Put it in a pan, add a bit of water and cook the potatoes for about 15 to 20 minutes. You need to make sure that the potatoes are not overcooked. Drain the potatoes and allow them to dry for a few minutes. Pour some olive oil in a pan, add the potatoes and cook over medium heat. Do not stir the potatoes. With the potatoes get crisp and golden on one side, turn it around gently so that it is same on both sides. Place these potatoes onto paper towels to allow them get rid of oil. Add lemon slice and cook until the sides are golden. Squeeze fresh lemon juice for some nice taste and the dish is ready to be savored.

Recipe 18: Honey and Dijon Potato Salad

A plate of potato salad serves as a huge boost in fighting headaches and migraines.

Ingredients:

- 3-4 potatoes
- 2-3 tablespoon olive oil
- ¼ cup apple cider vinegar
- ¼ cup whole grain Dijon mustard
- ½ finely diced red onion
- Honey, salt and pepper

Method:

Chop the potatoes into big 5-7 pieces and boil them in salted water. Make sure they are not overcooked as the dish will not taste better then. Drain and allow it to cool. Put olive oil, onion and garlic in a pan and allow it to warm over medium heat. Stir for a few minutes and then add the potatoes into the mixture. Toss the pan a few times till the potatoes get hot and well coated. Mix cider vinegar, honey, salt and pepper and the dish is ready to be served.

Recipe 19: Potato Soup

Though many people have not even heard of potato soup, forget tasting; potato soup is a quick and easy to make dish that can start working on your headache once taken.

Ingredients:

- 2 boiled potatoes
- 1 cup milk
- Garlic cloves
- 1 chopped onion and a few spring onions
- Salt and pepper

Method:

Boil the potatoes and mash it after peeling the skin. Add milk to it to arrive at a creamy and thick liquid. After that add some butter in a pan and sauté the sliced onions and garlic till the mixture is slightly brown. Add the potatoes and milk mixture to the pan. Allow it boil for a few minutes. To that add chopped spring onions along with salt and pepper. Cook for a few more minutes and the potato soup is ready to fight your headache.

Recipe 20: Mojo Potatoes

A Mojo Potato is mainly an afternoon dish post lunch. It helps to curb the growing menace of post lunch headache and is usually served with hot tea.

Ingredients:

- Potatoes
- ¼ teaspoon Cayenne pepper
- ½ teaspoon garlic powder
- 3 tablespoon milk
- Cooking oil
- 1 cup flour

Method:

Wash the potatoes, prick it lightly and steam it for 15 minutes. Allow the potatoes to cool and after that cut the potatoes in round slices. Meanwhile, start heating oil in a cooking pan for a few minutes. On the other hand, stir the mixture of flour, cayenne, garlic powder in a plate. Dredge potatoes in this mixture and place them in the pan for frying until it is crisp and golden. Place the potatoes on butter paper to allow the oil to be soaked and season it with a pinch of salt and pepper.

Recipe 21: Potato Pancakes

Have you ever had potato pancakes? Did you ever know that a dish like this exists and can help in bringing a relief from headache and migraine? Potato pancakes offer a rich source of potassium that can be served with a ginger iced tea.

Ingredients:

- 3-4 potatoes
- ¼ cup hot milk
- ½ cup grated carrots
- ¼ cup finely chopped onions and green onions
- 2 tablespoon flour
- 2 to 3 tablespoons cooking oil

Method:

Steam the potatoes for about 15 minutes. Take a pan and pour the milk. Mash the potatoes and add the mixture of carrots, onion, flour and milk in a mixing bowl. Form thick, large, circular balls that are a bit flat and bake them till they are golden brown. Garnish the pancake with grated carrots, salt and pepper.

Part 5: Lavender

Lavender has some wonderful soothing and calming properties that can bring your headache to cool down. Lavender aromatherapy is the most effective and widely prescribed therapy to cure migraines. It is said to be a great respite from any kind of headache.

Recipe 22: Lavender Roasted Potatoes

The combination of lavender and potatoes is extremely good when it comes to relieving pain caused due to migraines. The soothing properties of edible lavender and energy filled potatoes help a lot in calming you down from severe migraine attack.

Ingredients:

- 4-5 potatoes
- 2 tablespoon olive oil
- 1-2 tablespoon dried lavender
- Salt and Pepper

Method:

Cut the potatoes into bite size pieces after scrubbing out any bad spots. Keep the skin as it is. Toss the small pieces of potatoes in a bowl filled with olive oil. Add lavender to it. Roast the mixture for about 15 minutes or until the potatoes are evenly done. Add salt and pepper for better taste.

Recipe 23: Hot Lavender Tea

A hot cup of lavender tea helps in relieving and calming the headache.

Ingredients:

- 3 tbsp. fresh lavender flowers or 1 1/2 tbsp. dried lavender flowers
- 2 cups of boiling water
- Honey and lemon if desired

Method:

First, immerse the lavender flowers into a teapot containing the boiling water. Allow the flowers to soak for at least thirty minutes. This allows for a strong concentrate. You can then serve this tea into cups and add more hot water if you wish to make it less strong. Add honey or a squeeze of lemon if desired.

Recipe 24: Pink Lemonade Lavender Sorbet

Apart from cooling and thirst quenching, this sorbet also helps in reducing the pain caused due to headaches and migraines.

Ingredients:

- 1 cup of naturally flavored Pink Lemonade
- 1 teaspoon of dried culinary lavender
- 1 tablespoon citron-age
- Sugar

Method:

Put lemonade, lavender and sugar in a small pan. Heat the pan on a medium flame and keep stirring to dissolve the sugar. Do this for at least 5 – 10 minutes. Turn off the heat and allow it to cool. Once cooled, cover the mixture and refrigerate until chilled.

This sorbet tastes better in the summer where you need a drink that cools you down both physically and mentally.

Recipe 25: Lavender infused Oil

Try this lavender infused oil to inhale during aromatherapy to get the best results for calming your nerves during a stiff migraine attack.

Ingredients:

- Water
- Olive oil, almond oil or any other oil
- 5 tablespoons fresh lavender flowers or 6 tablespoons dried lavender flowers

Method:

Let the dried or fresh lavender flowers be infused in the oil in a jar, leaving some space above. Let it be immersed overnight and through an entire day, keeping it in contact with direct sunlight. The longer you steep the oil with the flowers, the more fragrant it will get.

Once done, strain the oil of the flowers using a muslin cloth or a cheese cloth or even a fine mesh strainer. To make the oil stronger, you can even add in a bunch of fresh lavender flowers and repeat the process.

To finish with, add a few drops of vitamin E at the end to help increase the shelf life of it. Use the oil as and when you please either to inhale in aromatherapy or to apply in small amounts.

Recipe 26: Lavender Honey Syrup

You can try the Lavender Honey Syrup twice or thrice in a day, depending upon the severity of the headache.

Ingredients:

- 1 cup honey
- ½ cup sugar
- 1 cup water
- ½ cup lavender flowers

Method:

Start boiling water and lavender in a saucepan. Add sugar and honey to the mixture and stir continuously till the sugar gets completely dissolved. Reduce the flame and allow the mixture to cool, strain and bottle. The mixture is then ready to be taken as and when desired.

Part 6: Salads

Salads are the most sensible thing to have if you want to lead a healthy life. Some salad recipes also prove to be helpful in bringing relief from migraine headaches. So lets have a look at some mouth watering salad recipes.

Recipe 27: Romaine and Smoked Salmon Salad

Salmon is known for omega 3 fatty acids which help in reducing the frequency of migraine attack. It also has strong anti-inflammatory properties which also contribute in preventing headaches.

Ingredients:

- 5 ounces of smoked salmon
- 1 organic romaine lettuce
- 2 tomatoes
- 4 radishes
- 1 carrot
- ½ peeled cucumber
- Lemon juice
- 1 tablespoon canola oil
- 1 tablespoon fresh ginger root

Method

Dice the tomatoes, slice radishes into thin pieces, diagonally slice the carrot, dice the cucumber and also thinly slice the salmon. Now arrange the lettuces on two plates and top it with salmon, tomatoes, radishes, carrots and cucumber. Pour the lemon juice, canola oil and minced ginger in a covered jar and shake it well. After that, pour the mixture over the salad. Your migraine reliever is ready to be served and tasted.

Recipe 28: Apple and Carrot Salad with Ginger

As simple as it sounds, this salad works best when migraine headaches attack you. It is a quick fire recipe that can be prepared in a quick span of time. Adding ginger to it makes it all the more tasty and helps in fighting a migraine attack.

Ingredients:

- 1 cup apple
- 1 cup carrot
- 2 tablespoons apple juice
- 1 tablespoon fresh ginger
- 2 tablespoons olive oil
- Lettuce leaves

Method:

Dice apple and carrot and put them in a small bowl. Mix apple juice, ginger and olive oil in a separate bowl and add to that diced apple and carrot. Toss it gently and you can serve on lettuce leaves or cut the leaves in small parts and can even add it as is to the salad.

Recipe 29: White Bean Asparagus Salad

Asparagus and beans are good to fight migraine and headaches.

Ingredients:

- 8-10 asparagus
- A bowl of whole beans
- 6 tomatoes
- ¼ cup fresh parsley
- ¼ cup vinegar
- 1 tablespoon olive oil
- 1 teaspoon Dijon mustard
- 1 teaspoon salt
- Black pepper

Method:

Take a saucepan and put some water to boil. Put the asparagus and allow it to steam for roughly around 3 to 5 minutes. Take the asparagus and allow it to cool. Take a wide bowl and combine the beans, tomatoes, parsley and cooled asparagus. Before that, you need to halve the tomatoes and chop the parsley. In a small bowl, mix vinegar, olive oil and mustard. Add salt and pepper to the mixture and whisk. Pour it over the bean salad and toss it gently.

Recipe 30: Grilled Salmon and Citrus Salad

Ingredients:

- 2 salmon fillets
- 2 cups baby spinach
- ½ orange
- ½ grapefruit
- ¼ cup red onions
- 1 tablespoon almonds
- 4-5 olives
- 2 tablespoons citrus vinaigrette
- 2 tablespoons soy sauce
- 1 tablespoon olive oil
- 1 teaspoon honey

Method:

Remove the skin of the fillets. Thinly slice the red onions and almonds. Take a large plastic bag and pour honey and soy sauce into the bag. Shake it well and add salmon. Ensure that it coats well and refrigerate for 10-15 minutes. Remove the salmon from the mixture and place it in a pan coated with olive oil. Discard the mixture of honey and sauce. Broil the pan until the fish is opaque. Take a bowl and mix spinach, orange and grapefruit, onion, almonds and olives. Top the bowl with a piece of fish and sprinkle citrus over it.

Recipe 31: Avocado Watermelon Spinach Salad

This is a completely delightful dish that is not only rich in taste, but also calms the nerves that are aching due to chronic migraine and headache.

Ingredients:

- 2 large avocados, peeled and diced
- 4 cups of cubed watermelon
- 4 cups of fresh spinach leaves
- Salt and pepper

Method:

Take a salad bowl and toss the above ingredients. Spray some salt and pepper and again toss so that it evenly applies to all the ingredients. Watermelon when served cold tastes best in this delicious salad dish.

Part 7: Juices and Smoothies

Who doesn't like to drink juices and smoothies? We all like it, isn't it? Juices and smoothies are a few of the best ways to reduce the pain caused due to migraines and headaches.

Recipe 32: The Green Juice

When attached with a severe migraine, the green juice is the one to have. It contains top three ingredients that help in curing headaches.

Ingredients:

- 1 cup pineapple
- 1 cup kale
- 1 cup cucumber
- Lemon juice
- Ginger
- Water and ice

Method:

Put all the above ingredients in a blender and process till it is smooth. This Green Juice will help in easing the trouble caused due to a migraine as pineapple contains bromelain, a natural enzyme for pain relief, ginger, which reduces inflammation, and cucumber that helps keep you hydrated.

Recipe 33: Green Breakfast

This juice is effective for eliminating headaches and migraines as the ingredients that are taken in this juice help in blocking the transmission of pain to a certain degree.

Ingredients:

- 2 apples
- 3 carrots
- 1 cucumber
- 1 cup grapes (green)
- 2 cups spinach
- 1 tomato

Method:

Process all the above mentioned ingredients in a juicer, shake it well and serve. You can add a tinge of honey for some sweetness.

Recipe 34: Veggie Blueberry

This broccoli rich juice, which is high in calcium and magnesium contains two essentials that help in fighting headaches and migraines.

Ingredients:

- 1 apple
- 1 cup blueberry
- 1 stalk broccoli
- 6 long carrots
- 1 whole tomato

Method:

Process all the ingredients in a juicer and shake well before serving.

Recipe 35: Fresh Salsa

Capsaicin in bell peppers along with celery blocks the transmission of pain to a certain level. Moreover the drink is highly nutritious and can help beat stress, fatigue and other ailments related to headache and migraine.

Ingredients:

- Cayenne pepper
- 1 stalk of large celery
- 1 cup of tomato cubes
- ½ tablespoon of garlic
- 1 medium sized spring onion
- Salt and pepper

Method:

Put all the ingredients in a blender and whip it well before serving.

Recipe 36: Carrot and Aloe Juice

Carrot and aloe juice is a blend of powerful and healthy juice to take on headaches.

Ingredients:

- 2 carrots
- 2 teaspoon of aloe juice
- Handful of alfalfa
- 1 teaspoon of liquid chlorophyll

Method:

Take all the above ingredients and blend it. Ensure that the mixture is not too thick. Else add some water. You can take this juice at lunchtime and will enhance the healing process of the headache.

Recipe 37: Banana Milkshake

Bananas are rich in Magnesium which helps in reducing the pain caused due to headaches as well as contains an ingredient called Tryptophan, which helps you to feel infinitely calm.

Ingredients:

- 5–6 ice cubes
- 1 medium-sized fresh banana
- 1/2 can of crushed pineapple
- Coconut essence or a tbsp. of shredded coconut
- ½ tsp. organic coconut oil

Method:

Begin by crushing the ice in the blender. Make sure that the ice is not completely crushed. Follow it up with the remaining ingredients. To give a subtle and refreshing twist to your milkshake, you can add cocoa powder and a tablespoon of instant coffee powder too.

Recipe 38: Watermelon Migraine Buster Smoothie

Watermelons are great to have, especially during summers. It is mainly because of the heat and dehydration that headaches occur and this watermelon smoothie helps to beat the headache in an apt way.

Ingredients:

- 2 cups of watermelon with seeds removed
- ½ peeled cucumber
- 1 tablespoon honey (if required)
- 2-3 mint leaves
- Ice

Method:

Add all the items in a blender and process it till it is smooth. You can add ice if the mixture gets too thin. It is best to serve with mint leaves on top of the glass.

Recipe 39: Grape and Green Smoothie

Apart from being rich in electrolytes and minerals, this smoothie is extremely rich in potassium and magnesium. These are two most vital elements that help beating headaches and migraines.

Ingredients:

- ¾ cup coconut water
- ¾ cup red grapes
- 1 banana
- 1 small cucumber
- 1 cup of spinach
- Ice

Method:

Wash all the ingredients well and chop cucumber and banana. Put these ingredients in a blender and blend it well. Pour over in a glass with ice cubes in it and enjoy! You can also substitute red grapes with a green one along with other fruits like strawberries or blueberries. Banana can be substituted with avocado, kiwi fruit, mango, lychee, or papaya.

Recipe 40: Avocado Smoothie

Avocado is known to be a stress buster as well as migraine shooter. Using it in this green colored smoothie helps in reducing migraine related headaches.

Ingredients:

- 1 cup coconut water
- 1 avocado
- 1 cup of frozen pineapple
- 1 tablespoon of grated fresh ginger
- 2 tablespoons of lime juice
- 1 scoop of vanilla protein powder

Method:

Put all the ingredients, except pineapple, in a blender and process it till the mixture is smooth. Afterwards, add pineapple and churn it a few times. Then process it until smooth.

Part 8: Cucumber

Cucumber is a vegetable with high water content that helps in reducing the headache and can hydrate the dehydrated body in minutes.

Recipe 41: Creamy Cucumber

Creamy cucumber is a delicious cucumber dish that one can have to ease the pain caused due to migraine.

Ingredients:

- 1 sliced cucumber
- Packaged cream cheese
- Packaged Italian salad dressing mix
- ½ cup mayonnaise
- 1 loaf of bread
- Pepper

Method:

Take a bowl and evenly mix cream cheese, mayonnaise and dressing mix. Cut the loaf into thick even pieces and spread a thin layer of just prepared cream cheese mixture over it. Place a slice of cucumber over the bread and sprinkle some pepper to enhance the taste.

Recipe 42: Cucumber and Avocado Sushi

A combination of cucumber and avocado to beat the summer heat as well as to cure the headache is your best bet when it comes to cucumber.

Ingredients:

- 1 cup sushi rice
- ½ cucumber, sliced into thin strips
- 1 peeled and sliced avocado
- 1 tablespoon rice vinegar
- Salt and pepper

Method:

Pour some water in a saucepan and add rice to it. Boil it for a few minutes and cover the pan. Reduce the heat after a few minutes and simmer for 15 to 20 minutes. Make sure that the rice is tender and the water is completely absorbed. Once the rice is tender, remove it from the pan and stir in vinegar. Add a pinch of salt while stirring. Allow the rice to cool.

Now, take a bamboo sushi mat and cover it with a plastic wrap to keep the rice from sticking. Spread rice evenly on it. Take cucumber and avocado and place it in the center of the rice. Now lift the mat and slowly roll it over and press. Your cucumber sushi is ready to be served!

Recipe 43: Cucumber Lemonade

An alternative to watermelon is cucumber and what better than having a cucumber lemonade to beat your headache?

Ingredients:

- 1 sliced cucumber
- Juices of 2 lemons
- White sugar

Method:

Place the saucepan filled with water and sugar. Keep stirring and heat it until it is just about to boil. Place the liquid in the refrigerator to cool. Now take the cucumber slices and blend it until it is mashed into a liquid form. Add water in case it is needed. Serve the syrup, cucumber liquid and lemon juice cold after stirring it well. You can add salt and pepper too.

Recipe 44: Cucumber Snack

Cucumber snack is an easy to make dish that is rich in nutritional value as well as helps in beating headaches and migraines.

Ingredients:

- 1 cucumber
- 2 tablespoon of low fat paneer
- 1 tablespoon freshly chopped dill leaves
- ½ tablespoon chilli paste
- 1 tablespoon low fat curd

Method:

Take the cucumber, peel it nicely and cut into two parts vertically. Dig out the center of each piece and keep them aside. Put the remaining ingredients in a bowl, mix it well and divide it into equal parts. Then stuff each cucumber slice with the prepared mixture. Cut each slice into equal parts and garnish it will dill leaves. This dish is to be served immediately.

Recipe 45: Cold Cucumber Soup

Have you ever had a soup that is not cold? Have you ever had a soup consisting of not the routine ingredients but cucumber? Well, if you want a relief from migraine then this cold cucumber soup can come to your rescue.

Ingredients:

- 1 cup of cucumber cubes
- ½ cup of finely chopped cucumber
- ½ cup low fat milk
- ¼ cup low fat curd
- 1 tablespoon finely chopped capsicum
- 2 tablespoons low fat butter

Method:

Put the cucumber cubes along with some amount of water in a saucepan and allow it to cook on a medium flame for 10 to 15 minutes. Make sure that the cucumber turns soft. Once it is done, allow the cucumber to cool. Take the cooled cucumber, milk, curd and salt and blend it till the mixture turns out to be smooth. Now heat the butter in another pan and add the chopped cucumber cubes, capsicum and sauté for 2 to 3 minutes. Once done, allow it to cool for a few minutes and mix the cucumber milk mixture to it and refrigerate. You can then serve this soup chilled and garnish it with mint leaves.

Part 9: Coffee

Coffee contains caffeine, which is a vasoconstrictor and it helps in alleviating a headache. However, care needs to be taken as too much intake of coffee can lead to more headaches instead of alleviating it.

Recipe 46: Spicy Coffee

This is a hot and spicy coffee whipped with cream to offer a perfect treat to your aching head.

Ingredients:

- A small cinnamon stick
- 1 clove
- 1-2 tablespoon sugar
- 1 tablespoon coffee powder

Method:

Mix all the above ingredients in a bowl and allow it to boil till the flavors start reaching towards you. Take the bowl off from the burner and allow it cool for a few minutes, not more than 5. Strain and pour into the cup and add 1 tablespoon whipped cream and a pinch of cinnamon to it.

Recipe 47: Chocolate Cinnamon Coffee

A spicy drink that is hot allows to calm yourself, de-stress and eases the pain caused due to headaches.

Ingredients:

- 1 tablespoon coffee powder
- 1 tablespoon whipped cream
- ½ cup of milk
- 1 tablespoon melted chocolate
- A pinch of nutmeg and cinnamon

Method:

Mix all the above ingredients excluding whipped cream in a cup. Take ½ cup of milk and allow it to boil. Once it starts boiling, pour over the mixture into the milk. Take it over and allow it to cool for a few minutes so that the flavors get infused. Top it with whipped cream and serve.

Recipe 48: Banana Coffee Frappe

Banana and coffee blend beautifully, thereby creating a strong drink, which can handle migraines and headaches. If you are into coffee, then this is the drink to go for to curb your headache.

Ingredients:

- 1 scoop of vanilla ice cream
- 1 tablespoon of coffee powder
- ½ banana, chopped

Method:

Mix all the above ingredients including some ice cubes together and blend it till the mixture is smooth and frothy.

Recipe 49: Coffee Walnut Smoothie

A combination of coffee and walnut serves well to fight headaches.

Ingredients:

- 1-2 tablespoon coffee powder
- ½ cup of walnut
- 1 tablespoon choco chips
- 2-3 drops of vanilla essence
- 3-4 tablespoon of honey

Method:

Mix all the ingredients and blend it till it is smooth. Pour into a serving glass and garnish it with mint leaves.

Recipe 50: Ginger Coffee

For all those who want to add some new taste, then go for ginger coffee. Not only it is good for curing headaches if taken on a daily basis, but also good for other ailments.

Ingredients:

- 1-2 tablespoon coffee powder
- Dried ginger
- 1-2 tablespoon of honey
- 5-8 peppercorns

Method:

Take a slightly deep vessel and add water, coffee powder, peppercorns and ginger to it. Allow the mixture to boil and reduce the flame when the water is reduced to half. Add a few drops of honey and a couple of mint leaves. Stir the mixture for couple of minutes. Strain and the coffee is ready to drink.

Conclusion

Headache disorder is highly common among people in today's time and a common type of nervous disorder. On an average, one out of three people in the world is said to suffer from tension types of headache (TTH) which is a scary statistic. The erratic work schedule and constant pressure to perform and deliver is leading people suffering from chronic headaches leading to migraines. From tensions to peer pressure, headaches have turned out to be nothing less than an enemy. People have forgotten how to relax and let go.

Headaches can occur due to medications too. Therefore, it is wise to avoid medication as much as possible, especially for headaches and migraines. Making the right lifestyle changes and taking in a little effort to create remedies from natural ingredients is the right way to do it.

After going through the pages of this book, you would have found yourself 50 easy remedies that can help you to beat headaches and migraines. These simple recipes throw light on what combination of ingredients you can use that not only suits you, but also help in eliminating the signs of headaches and migraines.

Made in the USA
Lexington, KY
17 July 2019